PANCREATIC SURGERY RECOVERY DIET

Empowering Your Healing Journey And Revitalizing Your Health For Surgery Recovery

DR LUCAS KAYCE

DISCLAIMER

This book about illness and nutrition is not meant to replace expert medical advice, diagnosis, or treatment; rather, it is meant purely for informational reasons. This book's content is founded on broad concepts and recommendations for managing diseases and nutrition.

Before adopting any major dietary or lifestyle changes, readers are recommended to speak with a qualified healthcare provider, such as a licensed physician or registered dietitian, especially if they have pre-existing medical concerns. Everybody has different health demands, so what works for one person might not work for another.

The use of the information provided in this book may have unfavorable repercussions or consequences, for which the author and publisher disclaim all liability. No disease is meant to be identified, treated, cured, or prevented by the information provided.

The book may include contain references to medical literature or research findings; however readers are urged to independently confirm this material and contact reliable sources.

It is important to remember that the fields of nutrition and medicine are always changing, and that new findings could have an impact on the advice offered in this book. As a result, readers are urged to keep up with the most recent advancements in healthcare and, when in doubt, seek professional counsel.

By reading this book, readers agree that they are in charge of their own health decisions and release the author and publisher from any liability arising from the use of the material in the book, whether direct or indirect.

TABLE OF CONTENTS

ABOUT THE BOOK

For those who have had pancreatic surgery, the book "Pancreatic Surgery Recovery Diet" tackles a crucial part of their recovery journey. One cannot stress the need for a customized recovery diet because the difficulties and dietary requirements following these procedures are distinct and rigorous.

An overview of pancreatic surgery is given at the outset of the thorough investigation, along with information on the various procedures and typical causes for undergoing them. Readers must grasp this background information to comprehend the next chapters.

The importance of diet in the healing process is one of the book's key topics. The importance of a healthy diet is explored in detail in the second chapter, which also highlights the direct impact of nutrition on healing and rehabilitation. It outlines the dietary issues that patients may have following surgery. The book then provides helpful advice in the form of post-surgery dietary suggestions, which advance from a time of a clear liquid diet to a gradual reintroduction of solid foods.

The book shifts its emphasis to foods high in nutrients that promote healing, going beyond the first few days following surgery. The role that protein, healthy fats and oils, complex carbohydrates, and vital vitamins and minerals play in the healing process is discussed in detail. Managing digestive symptoms, such as nausea, diarrhea, and constipation, is important to take into account. Useful advice is offered to enhance digestion in general.

Understanding that every patient is unique, the book discusses how to tailor the recovery diet to meet particular demands. Personalized meal planning, adjusting to dietary restrictions, and the significance of consulting a trained dietician are all part of this. Creating a supportive environment, recognizing the emotional aspects of treatment, and including family and friends in the process are all examples of the holistic approach.

The book highlights the sustainability of constructive modifications by including chapters on long-term lifestyle modifications. The need for follow-up treatment and monitoring, adding regular physical activity, and keeping a balanced diet beyond recovery are just a few of the insightful information that readers will discover. The book ends with a compilation of breakfast, lunch, dinner, snack, and dessert dishes that are specially designed to aid in the recuperation from pancreatic surgery. This helps to further simplify the actual application of the knowledge. All things considered, "Pancreatic Surgery Recovery Diet" is an invaluable manual that offers advice as well as doable actions for fruitful and long-lasting recuperation.

AN OVERVIEW OF SURGERY ON THE PANCREAS

At the vanguard of contemporary medical interventions is pancreatic surgery, which includes a range of procedures intended to treat different pancreatic problems. Surgery may be necessary to treat a variety of conditions affecting the pancreas, an essential organ that produces insulin and digestive enzymes, including tumors, cysts, and chronic pancreatitis.

Because pancreatic surgery is such a delicate and intricate procedure, it requires a multidisciplinary team of experienced surgeons, anesthesiologists, and specialist nurses. These treatments, which are specifically designed to treat particular diseases and improve patient outcomes, may include distal pancreatectomy, total pancreatectomy, and pancreaticoduodenectomy (also known as the Whipple procedure).

A customized recovery diet plays a crucial part in the postoperative recovery process, which is one of the key factors influencing the success of pancreatic surgery. It is imperative to stress the critical role that a customized nutrition plan plays in facilitating healing, addressing problems, and enhancing the general well-being of patients during the recovery phase. Following pancreatic surgery, a customized recovery diet is created to address the particular dietary requirements and difficulties that individuals encounter while they heal. The goal of this diet is to facilitate a smoother transition to a healthy postoperative life by managing digestive changes, supplying important nutrients, and lowering the risk of problems.

THE VALUE OF A CUSTOMIZED REHAB DIET

A thorough awareness of the several surgical procedures used and the underlying problems that require such interventions is necessary to navigate the complexities of pancreatic surgery. To handle the complexity of the pancreas, surgeons who specialize in pancreatic treatments need to have a thorough understanding of its anatomy, pathology, and cutting-edge surgical techniques. Robotic-assisted surgeries and minimally invasive procedures are becoming more common as technology continues to change the surgical intervention landscape. These methods promise shorter recovery times and better patient outcomes.

Advances in surgery are not enough to overshadow the significance of a customized recovery diet. The unique difficulties that come with pancreatic surgery—such as altered digestive function, possible malabsorption problems, and the requirement for sufficient nutritional support—are addressed by a well-organized postoperative diet plan. This nutritional strategy not only speeds up the healing process but also lowers the chance of side effects from pancreatic surgery, like gastrointestinal distress and malnourishment.

A study of pancreatic surgery uncovers a specialty at the nexus of cutting-edge medicine, skill in surgery, and comprehensive patient care.

Patients and healthcare providers alike must comprehend the subtleties of various pancreatic treatments and their repercussions. Concurrently, recognizing the critical function of a customized recovery diet highlights the significance of a comprehensive strategy for postoperative care. With the advancement of medical technology, the combination of nutritional support and surgical accuracy has the potential to completely change the field of pancreatic surgery and improve the lives of those who need these complex procedures.

CHAPTER ONE

COMPREHENDING PANCREATIC SURGERY

PANCREATIC SURGERY TYPES

A variety of techniques, each catered to the unique requirements of the patient, is included in pancreatic surgery and is intended to treat different pancreatic ailments. The Whipple technique, sometimes referred to as pancreaticoduodenectomy, is a popular and complex kind of pancreatic surgery. The pancreatic head, the gallbladder, the duodenum, a section of the stomach, and the surrounding lymph nodes are all removed during this procedure. After that, the remaining organs are rebuilt to aid in digestion and preserve regular body processes.

Distal pancreatectomy is another kind of pancreatic surgery in which the pancreas's body and tail are removed. When a condition or cancer is restricted to the lower portion of the pancreas, this surgery is frequently carried out. Furthermore, although a total pancreatectomy has major long-term ramifications for the patient's digestive health, it may be advised in circumstances where the condition is so severe that the entire pancreas must be removed.

TYPICAL INDICATIONS FOR PANCREAS SURGERY

Although the causes of pancreatic surgery can vary, they frequently have to do with treating cystic neoplasms, pancreatitis, or pancreatic cancer. Because of its aggressive nature, pancreatic cancer may require surgery to remove the tumor and any damaged tissues. Surgery may be necessary to treat pancreatitis, an inflammation of the pancreas, if nonsurgical measures are ineffective or if complications including pseudocysts and abscesses develop.

Fluid-filled sacs on or inside the pancreas called cystic neoplasms may also need to be surgically removed if they provide a considerable risk of cancer or produce symptoms.

GETTING READY FOR SURGERY

A comprehensive evaluation and collaboration between the patient, surgical team, and other medical specialists are necessary while preparing for pancreatic surgery. Preoperative assessments usually consist of a thorough medical history, a physical examination, and different imaging tests to ascertain the severity of the pancreatitis. Patients may also have electrocardiograms, blood tests, and other evaluations to make sure they are healthy enough to have surgery.

Patients are routinely informed on the possible dangers, advantages, and outcomes of pancreas surgery to help them prepare psychologically. It is stressed how crucial it is to follow preoperative instructions, such as fasting before surgery and stopping specific drugs.

In addition, patients can consult with an anesthesiologist to go over the anesthetic strategy and ask any questions they may have about the process.

Having the support of friends and family and keeping lines of communication open with the medical staff is essential during the preoperative period. By working together, we can make sure that patients are psychologically and physically ready for pancreatic surgery, which improves the procedure's overall outcome and patients' ability to recover afterward.

CHAPTER TWO

THE FUNCTION OF DIET IN THE RECOVERY AFTER PANCREATIC SURGERY

THE VALUE OF A BALANCED DIET

Following pancreatic surgery, patients' recovery is greatly aided by proper diet, which is essential for their general health and recuperation. It is impossible to exaggerate how crucial it is to keep up a healthy diet because it has a direct impact on the body's capacity to recover from surgery, restore strength, and avoid complications.

In the context of recovering from pancreatic surgery, a well-balanced and nutrient-rich diet is especially important for boosting the body's immune system, encouraging tissue healing, and lowering the risk of infection.

NUTRITIONAL DIFFICULTIES FOLLOWING SURGERY

After pancreatic surgery, nutritional issues frequently surface, posing special problems because of the pancreas' complex role in digestion and metabolism. The possible reduction of pancreatic enzyme synthesis, which is crucial for nutrient absorption and digestion, is one major problem. This may result in problems with malabsorption, which could impair the body's capacity to absorb vital vitamins, minerals, and other nutrients from meals. As a result, patients can be deficient in important components like certain minerals and fat-soluble vitamins (A, D, E, and K), which would call for particular dietary changes and, occasionally, supplementation.

EFFECTS ON RECUPERATION AND HEALING

Adequate diet has a significant impact on the healing and recuperation process following pancreatic surgery. Sufficient consumption of nutrients is directly related to the body's capacity to mend tissues, lessen inflammation, and regain vigor. In particular, protein becomes essential since it helps maintain muscular mass and promotes the growth of new tissues. Protein-based essential amino acids play a major role in the healing process by aiding in the reconstruction of injured cells and tissues.

Nutrition is also a major factor in the management of problems following surgery. Patients having pancreas surgery could be more susceptible to infections, and a healthy body is better able to fight off any invaders. Furthermore, a healthy diet can help reduce the risk of postoperative complications such as infections, gastrointestinal problems, and delayed wound healing. A body in proper nutritional condition is more resilient, which facilitates a quicker recovery and shortens hospital stays overall.

It is impossible to overestimate the significance of diet for the healing process following pancreatic surgery. To manage the special difficulties that follow surgery, promote the body's healing processes, and reduce the chance of problems, proper nutrition is crucial. An effective nutritional plan that is customized to meet the unique requirements of patients recuperating from pancreatic surgery is an essential component of total patient care and greatly enhances prognosis and quality of life.

CHAPTER THREE

POST-OPERATIVE NUTRITIONAL
GUIDELINES

THE PHASE OF CLEAR LIQUID DIET

Following certain dietary recommendations is essential for a speedy recovery following surgery. The Clear Liquid Diet Phase is one of the first stages of post-surgery dietary instructions. Drinking translucent, easily digestible beverages is a hallmark of this phase. transparent liquids include transparent fruit juices, gelatin, broth, and water. The goal of this stage is to supply vital nutrients and hydration without taxing the digestive system. It is frequently recommended that patients move on to this stage as soon as they can take fluids and are not suffering any nausea or vomiting.

MAKING THE SWITCH TO A SOFT DIET

The next critical stage in the post-surgery dietary path is switching to a Soft Diet. During this stage, meals that are higher in fat and nutrients can be added without negatively impacting the digestive system. Pureed fruits and vegetables, yogurt, oatmeal, and well-cooked mashed potatoes are examples of soft foods. The objective of this stage is to ease the transition from liquid to solid foods by progressively reintroducing a range of nutrients and textures. It's critical to consider each person's tolerance level and proceed at a rate that corresponds with the body's capacity to process increasingly complicated foods.

INTRODUCING SOLID FOODS GRADUALLY

The last stage of the post-surgery dietary guidelines, the Gradual Introduction of Solid Foods, represents a critical turning point in the healing process. Patients can begin including a greater variety of solid foods in their diet during this period, with an emphasis on nutrient-dense selections. Lean proteins, whole grains, fruits, and vegetables may be examples of this. But it's important to proceed cautiously during this stage, introducing one kind of solid food at a time and keeping an eye on the body's reaction.

To prevent overtaxing the digestive system during this phase, doctors frequently advise smaller, more frequent meals.

Maintaining regular contact with healthcare specialists and following personalized suggestions are crucial during these dietary periods. It is necessary to take into account variables such as the kind of surgery, the patient's general health, and any particular dietary requirements. A common theme throughout all phases is remaining well-hydrated since sustaining appropriate bodily processes and promoting general recovery depend on consuming enough fluids. All things considered, the process of moving through these nutritional phases is progressive and individualized, guaranteeing a supportive and well-rounded approach to nutrition following surgery.

CHAPTER FOUR

RICH IN NUTRIENT FOODS FOR RECUPERATION

FOODS HIGH IN PROTEIN

Proteins are essential for the healing process, particularly following strenuous exercise or physical exertion. They support the healing of injured tissues and serve as the building blocks of muscles. You must include meals high in protein in your diet if you want to support general wellness and muscle recovery. Lean meats like turkey, chicken, and fish, as well as plant-based foods like beans, lentils, and tofu, are good sources of high-quality protein. Dairy products, eggs, and nuts can also help you consume the amount of protein required for the best possible recuperation.

NUTRITIOUS FATS AND OILS

Healthy fats are essential for healing and general health, despite the common misunderstanding that they should be avoided. Omega-3 fatty acids, which are present in walnuts, flaxseeds, and fatty fish like salmon and trout, have anti-inflammatory qualities that can help lessen inflammation and discomfort in the muscles after a workout.

Rich in monounsaturated fats, which assist the body's healing process and offer a source of sustained energy, are almonds, avocados, and olive oil. Including these beneficial fats in your diet aids in preserving the proper ratio of vital nutrients for faster healing.

COMPLEX GLYCOSOMICS

The main source of energy is carbohydrates, and eating complex carbs is essential to refueling the glycogen stores that are used up during physical exercise. Brown rice, quinoa, and oats are examples of whole grains that are great providers of complex carbs that release energy gradually. In addition to providing vital fiber and useful carbs, sweet potatoes, legumes, and fruits also facilitate nutrient absorption and digestion. Including these complex carbs in your post-workout meals encourages the body to restore its glycogen stores and facilitates faster recovery.

VITAL MINERALS AND VITAMINS

Minerals and vitamins are essential for many physiological functions, such as healing and immunological response. Berries and citrus fruits are rich sources of vitamin C, which promotes the synthesis of collagen and aids in the healing of connective tissues. Vitamin D is necessary for healthy bones and general well-being. It can be gained from sunshine exposure and some meals, such as fatty fish. Nuts, bananas, and leafy green vegetables are good sources of minerals including magnesium and potassium, which support electrolyte balance and muscle performance. Having a varied and nutrient-rich diet aids in fulfilling the body's needs for these vital vitamins and minerals, fostering the best possible healing and general well-being.

The key to assisting the body's healing process is to concentrate on eating a well-balanced, nutrient-rich diet that contains enough protein, healthy fats, complex carbs, and vital vitamins and minerals. By incorporating these components into your diet, you may enhance general health, minimize inflammation, and facilitate muscle repair more quickly, which will help you reach your fitness goals and recover as quickly as possible.

CHAPTER FIVE

HANDLING SYMPTOMS OF DIGESTION

HANDLING SEIZURES

Common stomach symptoms like nausea can be brought on by several things, such as prescription drugs, food choices, or underlying medical disorders. Finding the source of the nausea and taking appropriate action to address it are essential. If your nausea is caused by a particular food allergy or intolerance, you may feel better if you cut certain foods out of your diet. Teas infused with ginger, peppermint, and chamomiles have anti-nausea qualities and can be drunk to ease upset stomachs. Since dehydration can worsen the symptoms, eating smaller, more frequent meals and maintaining hydration can also help manage nausea.

TREATING CONSTIPATION AND DIARRHEA

Constipation and diarrhea both have a substantial negative influence on a person's quality of life and treating both gastrointestinal disorders requires specialized care. Maintaining hydration is crucial for replacing lost fluids and electrolytes when experiencing diarrhea. The BRAT diet, which consists of basic, easily digested meals like toast, applesauce, rice, and bananas, can help settle the stomach.

Reducing your intake of dairy, coffee, high-fat, and spicy meals can all help with symptom relief. To rule out underlying illnesses, it is essential to consult a physician if diarrhea persists.

On the other side, dietary and lifestyle changes are frequently effective in treating constipation. Regular bowel movements are encouraged by increasing the amount of fiber consumed through the diet by including whole grains, fruits, and vegetables.

Drinking enough water is important since fiber helps to absorb water and soften feces. Frequent exercise also aids in promoting bowel motions. While prolonged usage of over-the-counter laxatives should be monitored by a healthcare provider to avoid reliance, they may be taken into consideration.

SUGGESTIONS FOR ENHANCING DIGESTION

Developing behaviors that facilitate the effective breakdown and absorption of nutrients is part of optimizing digestion. Chewing food well is an easy but important step since it starts the digestive process in the mouth.

The body's capacity to concentrate on digestion can be improved by eating in a calm setting and minimizing distractions. Probiotics, which are present in fermented foods like sauerkraut and yogurt, help to maintain a balanced population of gut bacteria, which improves digestion.

Digestive health can also benefit from stress management practices including yoga, meditation, and deep breathing.

Furthermore, maintaining hydration throughout the day facilitates food digestion and passage through the digestive system. Being aware of your body's signals of hunger and fullness might help you avoid overindulging and maintain a healthy digestive tract. It's crucial to remember that everyone reacts differently to dietary modifications, and speaking with a healthcare provider can offer specific advice for successfully treating digestive difficulties.

CHAPTER SIX

TAILORING THE DIET TO EACH PERSON'S NEEDS

CUSTOMIZED FOOD SCHEDULE

Personalized meal planning is adjusting food selections to meet the specific requirements, tastes, and health objectives of each individual. This method takes into account many aspects like age, gender, activity level, and underlying health concerns, acknowledging that diets that are designed to accommodate all individuals may not be beneficial for everyone. People can maximize their nutritional intake and make sure they get the proper ratio of calories, macronutrients, and micronutrients by personalizing their meal plans.

GETTING USED TO PARTICULAR DIETARY RESTRICTIONS

A crucial component of tailoring diets to each person's requirements is adjusting to specific dietary restrictions. A lot of people are limited in what they can eat because of allergies, intolerances, or health issues. For instance, a person with celiac disease must avoid gluten-containing meals, but a person with lactose sensitivity may need to avoid dairy products. Tailored meal planning considers these limitations and offers options and replacements to guarantee a satisfying and well-rounded diet without sacrificing health or dietary needs.

MEETING WITH A NUTRITIONIST

Customizing diets for individual needs requires consultation with a dietitian. Dietitians are qualified experts who develop individualized nutrition regimens by evaluating each person's food preferences, lifestyle, and state of health. Dietitians can address individual concerns, educate patients about nutrition, and provide workable solutions for reaching dietary objectives in one-on-one appointments. To make the customization process more comprehensive, these experts also take into account psychological, social, and cultural aspects that may have an impact on dietary choices.

Dietitians work with clients to establish attainable dietary objectives during consultations. They may also keep an eye on developments over time and make modifications as necessary. A supportive and empowering relationship between the patient and the dietician is fostered by this individualized approach, which results in long-lasting dietary habit improvements. Dietitians improve adherence to dietary regimens by customizing suggestions to each patient's needs, which improves overall health results.

Personalized meal planning can take into account individual preferences, such as cooking skills, taste preferences, and cultural influences, in addition to dietary limitations. This guarantees that the personalized diet is long-lasting, pleasurable, and sufficiently nutrient-rich. Incorporating foods that people like and are accustomed to eating increases the likelihood that they will stick to the diet plan, which helps them reach their overall wellness and health objectives.

The notion of tailoring diets to individual requirements includes developing customized meal plans, adjusting to certain dietary constraints, and seeking advice from a nutritionist. This methodology acknowledges the individuality of every person's nutritional needs and endeavors to develop a dietary plan that is both sustainable and efficacious. People can get a customized diet that fits their lifestyle and health objectives by working with a nutritionist and taking into account several criteria.

CHAPTER SEVEN

CREATING A HELPFUL ENVIRONMENT

VALUE OF EMOTIONAL SUPPORT

Establishing a conducive atmosphere is crucial for people dealing with a range of difficulties, particularly when it comes to their health and overall well. Emotional support is one of the main tenets of this kind of care, and it is essential for building resilience and facilitating the healing process. It is impossible to exaggerate the significance of emotional support because it has a profound impact on one's mental and emotional health. Others' compassion, understanding, and support can ease stress, lessen anxiety, and improve one's general quality of life when dealing with health concerns.

FRIENDS AND FAMILY INVOLVEMENT

Having friends and family involved is essential to creating a nurturing atmosphere. These connections provide a strong support system of kindness and caring for people confronting health issues. Family members' presence creates a feeling of safety and acceptance, which promotes a healing environment. In addition to providing helpful advice and emotional support, family and friends provide a comprehensive support network that attends to the mental and physical needs of the individual.

ADAPTIVE TECHNIQUES FOR PATIENTS

A supportive atmosphere must include coping mechanisms, especially for people who are experiencing health problems. These techniques enable people to successfully negotiate obstacles, control their stress, and adjust to changing circumstances.

A nurturing atmosphere fosters the creation and application of coping strategies customized to meet the specific requirements of every person. This could entail practicing mindfulness, taking part in therapeutic activities, or getting help from a counselor. People can face health issues with resilience and optimism when they are in a supportive atmosphere that encourages and welcomes coping mechanisms.

Moreover, the significance of communication in a nurturing atmosphere cannot be disregarded. Understanding a patient's unique requirements and preferences requires open and honest communication between the patient, their healthcare providers, and their support system.

By facilitating information sharing, healthcare providers can adopt a collaborative approach to patient care, where choices are made jointly and the patient's voice is heard. A shared responsibility for well-being and the ability to actively participate in health management are two benefits of effective communication that enhance a person's sense of empowerment.

The establishment of a supportive environment includes the use of coping mechanisms, the provision of emotional support, and the participation of family and friends for those who are dealing with health issues.

This holistic approach recognizes the psychological and emotional facets of health in addition to the physical ones. Healing, resilience, and general well-being can be effectively catalyzed in a supportive atmosphere by cultivating empathy, understanding, and proactive coping skills.

CHAPTER EIGHT

LONG-TERM MODIFICATIONS TO LIFESTYLE

SUSTAINING A NUTRITIONAL PLAN AFTER REHABILITATION

Maintaining a nutritious diet is essential for long-term health as well as during the healing process. After the initial stages of recovery, people are urged to take up nutritional practices that enhance general well-being and stave off health problems from returning. Maintaining healthy body functions requires a diet rich in vital nutrients, including vitamins, minerals, and fiber, and balanced. It is essential to prioritize a range of dietary groups, such as whole grains, fruits, vegetables, lean meats, and healthy fats.

Moreover, portion management is essential to maintaining a balanced diet. By practicing moderation and paying attention to one's body's signals, one can avoid overindulging and promote general well-being and weight management.

A long-lasting and healthy connection with food is facilitated by using mindful eating techniques, such as enjoying every mouthful and being aware of your body's signals of hunger and fullness.

INCLUDING FREQUENT PHYSICAL EXERCISE

A healthy lifestyle is based on regular physical activity, which goes well beyond recovery times. Regular physical activity enhances mental health in addition to maintaining physical condition. People are advised to engage in activities they enjoy increasing the likelihood that they will incorporate exercise into their everyday lives and achieve long-term success.

Exercise routines that are in line with individual tastes and health objectives are crucial, whether they involve strength training exercises or cardiovascular exercises like cycling, jogging, or walking. Frequent exercise has several advantages, such as better weight management, improved mood and mental clarity, and cardiovascular health. A comprehensive approach to fitness can also be promoted by including flexibility and balance exercises, which can improve general mobility and lower the chance of injury.

MONITORING AND AFTERCARE

Following the initial phases of rehabilitation, monitoring, and follow-up care are essential parts of an all-encompassing healthcare plan. Visiting medical specialists regularly aids in monitoring the patient's development, spotting possible issues, and modifying the treatment plan as needed. Keeping an eye on health indicators like blood pressure, cholesterol, and other pertinent metrics guarantees that any departures from the intended range are quickly corrected.

In addition to routine checkups, people should take an active role in managing their health by learning about their diseases and realizing the value of preventive care. This could entail changing one's lifestyle, taking prescription drugs as directed, and identifying warning indicators for prompt action.

CHAPTER NINE

RECIPES FOR RECOVERING AFTER
PANCREATIC SURGERY

IDEAS FOR BREAKFAST

When recovering from pancreatic surgery, it's critical to focus on a nutrient-dense, readily-digested breakfast to start the day. Make healthy yet easy meals like oatmeal with cut berries or bananas. Soluble fiber from oats helps with digestion, while vitamins and minerals from fruits are also important.

Scrambled eggs are another healthy choice; they are high in protein and aid in muscle repair. You can add soft-cooked veggies, like bell peppers or spinach, to improve the nutritional value and flavor. A small portion of avocado or whole-grain bread can be a great way to add healthy fats and long-lasting energy to the meal.

Smoothies with low-fat yogurt, spinach, and a variety of fruits, such as mango and berries, can be a pleasant and nutrient-rich choice for people looking for something lighter. This offers hydration and several vitamins that are essential for the healing process.

RECIPES FOR LUNCH AND DINNER

During the recuperation period following pancreatic surgery, balanced meals that are easy on the digestive tract should be the focus of lunch and dinner. The foundation of these meals is a lean protein source, such as fish, tofu, or baked or grilled chicken. For long-lasting energy, combine it with simple-to-digest carbohydrates like sweet potatoes, brown rice, or quinoa.

Carrots, zucchini, and green beans are examples of vegetables that provide vital vitamins without taxing the digestive system when they are steamed or cooked briefly. Post-operative inflammation can be lessened by including anti-inflammatory herbs like turmeric or ginger.

Meals that are based on soup, such as homemade chicken or vegetable broth, can be calming and gentler on the stomach. To add extra nutrition, make sure the soup has a variety of vegetables. Incorporating healthy grains such as barley or couscous can improve the nutritional composition and offer a satisfying consistency.

DESSERTS AND SNACKS

During the recovery period following pancreatic surgery, snacking is essential for sustaining energy levels. Choose easily digested foods like a handful of nuts and seeds or Greek yogurt with a honey drizzle. These contribute to a balanced diet by offering a mix of healthy fats and protein.

Fresh fruits with natural sweetness and nutrition, such as berries, pears, or apples, make great snacks. Fruit can be combined with nut butter or a tiny amount of cheese to enhance flavor and increase protein content.

Make sure to select desserts that are easy on the digestive tract. Sweet tooths can be satiated with a fruit salad flavored with a little cinnamon or a baked apple topped with nutmeg, both of which won't interfere with the healing process after surgery.

It's important to drink enough water during all meals and snacks. During the healing phase, drinking lots of water throughout the day promotes healthy digestion and general well-being. Additionally, to ensure a smooth and healthy recovery following pancreatic surgery, speaking with a certified dietitian or healthcare expert can assist in customizing these meal suggestions to specific nutritional needs.